Natural Family Planning
Why It Succeeds

Second Edition

Herbert F. Smith S.J.

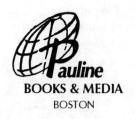

BOOKS & MEDIA

BOSTON

Imprimi Potest:
James A. Devereux, SJ
Provincial Superior

Nihil Obstat:
James McGrath
Censor Librorum

Imprimatur:
John Cardinal Krol
Archbishop of Philadelphia

ISBN 0-8198-5115-9

Printed and published in the U.S.A. by Pauline Books & Media, 50 Saint Pauls Avenue, Boston MA 02130-3491.

www.pauline.org

Pauline Books & Media is the publishing house of the Daughters of St. Paul, an international congregation of women religious serving the Church with the communications media.

2 3 4 5 6 7   04 03 02 01 00 99

Contents

1. Is Natural Family Planning (NFP) the best method of family planning? What is the evidence?

The best method is the one that achieves its purpose at the lowest cost. It's certain that Natural Family Planning (NFP) is the best method of family planning in many respects.

NFP is the safest method. It is non-invasive. It requires no drugs, no bodily inserts, no sterilization and no doctors. It does no harm to the body or the fertility of either partner, and yet it involves both. It does no harm to any offspring.

NFP is the fairest method. Other methods require one partner, usually the woman, to bear the whole burden of fertility control. In NFP, marriage partners share the burden.

NFP is a wholly natural method. It uses the mind to acquire fertility awareness, and uses the free will to govern conduct accordingly. It requires periods of sexual abstinence, but does not interfere in the act of intercourse. It maintains both intimacy and pleasure. In fact, the knowledge of biological characteristics gained in learning NFP can heighten a couple's intimacy.

NFP is family planning in the truest sense. Natural and wholesome, it serves at one time to plan conception and at another to exclude it. With NFP, high fertility couples can space and limit children; low fertility couples can enhance the hope of child-bearing by timing intercourse to the days of optimum fertility.

NFP is a scientific method. Properly learned, it is a reliable method of family planning. Because of its many positive side effects, it is proving to be a better method than anyone dreamed. An article on NFP in a national magazine ended with the remark, "Who knows? In a few years, the clunker of family planning methods may well end up a Cadillac" (*Insight*, April 14, 1986).

It is the least expensive method. After a small outlay to learn it, NFP costs almost nothing.

NFP is a method that is morally and religiously acceptable, provided that it is not used selfishly. It shines brightest in the area of deepest values. It harms neither conscience nor faith, neither reason nor one's relationship with God. For many people, these reasons tip the scale.

NFP contributes to a solution of four major world problems of our day: abortion, fear of a population explosion, moral and family disintegration from the contraceptive mentality, and religious breakdown with its attendant rebellion against Church authority. In that limited sense NFP is "the hundred percent solution," as I called it in an earlier pamphlet.

Without doctors, drugs or devices, couples can now teach one another fertility awareness and control, and grow in the process. NFP resolves the problem of regulating births in a wholesome way.

2. Is NFP genuinely new? How does it differ from the old rhythm method so many couples abandoned when the pill arrived?

Modern NFP is new. It is the breakthrough by which a woman becomes so knowledgeable about her own body that she knows the days on which she is fertile and can conceive.

Author of *The Ovulation Method Of Birth Control*, worldwide NFP teacher Mercedes Wilson described NFP at a

Catholic Physicians' Guild meeting in Philadelphia. She held the audience spellbound with her explanation of new scientific findings, fortified by charts and statistical evaluations of their effectiveness.

When she finished, some of the women who were present challenged her with an angry query, "Why haven't we been told of this method?" Let the media, the clergy and the doctors ponder that question.

The author explained NFP to a group of older men who were familiar with the old calendar rhythm method. They were quite skeptical. One old man's challenge rang of the adage, "Don't confuse me with the facts! I've made up my mind."

The author bided his time as if playing a cat and mouse game, trump card close to the vest. At last he played it—a pictorial chart. It showed the various patterns of cervical mucus in color. Properly understood, they reveal when a woman's fertile phase is approaching, and when it has passed. The old man who had been so hard to convince whispered in the author's ear, "That *is* different!"

Both cervical mucus and physical changes in the cervix signal first the approach of fertility, and then the receding of fertility. Further, a rise in the woman's body temperature indicates that ovulation has occurred. Then a woman can accurately judge when she will be infertile again.

The mucus or temperature can be used separately or as a cross-check for family planning. The cervical sign is a third cross-check. Guided by this information, the couple can plan intercourse to exclude or to achieve conception, as they wish.

To bring this into focus, let us compare the definition of modern NFP with that of the old calendar rhythm method. **Calendar rhythm** is family planning in which the fertile period is *estimated*, by a formula which relies on previous cycle lengths, to *predict* the limits of the present fertile time. Intercourse is timed to exclude or achieve conception in accord with this *estimate* of the fertile period.

Modern NFP

The World Health Organization's definition of NFP is: "Natural Family Planning: methods for planning or preventing pregnancies by observation of the naturally occurring signs and symptoms of the fertile and infertile phases of the menstrual cycle. It is implicit in the definition of NFP, when used to avoid conception, that drugs, devices and surgical procedures are not used; there is abstinence from sexual intercourse during the fertile phase of the menstrual cycle; and the act of sexual intercourse, when occurring, is complete."

These two definitions indicate the following differences in the methods: calendar rhythm relies on a *formula* which uses no input from the woman's body in the present cycle. It predicts the length of the present cycle from the length of past cycles.

NFP relies on a woman directly observing her fertility signs. The method is attuned to her body *here and now*. She "sees" each cycle unfolding phase by phase.

That explains why modern NFP is so reliable. Unlike the old rhythm system, it monitors each cycle. It works even in cycles which vary greatly in length, such as after childbirth, during breast-feeding, premenopause, etc.

Although NFP uses the rhythms of the cycle, it does so in a manner so different and superior to the old rhythm method that a new name had to be coined for it: Natural Family Planning. (It should be added that in all natural methods, including calendar rhythm, there is another common factor: during the fertile period, intercourse is engaged in to achieve conception, and abstained from to exclude conception.)

3. Would you give a more detailed explanation of how NFP works, and why it is better than the old rhythm method?

The surest way to understand NFP is to get an overview of the medical developments which led first to calendar rhythm and then to modern NFP.

Until this century, little was known of the menstrual cycle. In fact, doctors thought that menstruation and ovulation coincided. That false idea blighted any possibility of NFP.

Light came in 1923-24 when Dr. Kyusaku Ogino of Japan published the results of his research. He had discovered that ovulation occurs between the 12th and 16th day *before* menstruation. He also knew that cycle lengths vary.

He knew he had found a natural method of family planning, for once the fertile times of the cycle are known, so are the infertile times. Calendar rhythm was being born. In the words of NFP adviser Dr. Rudolf Vollman, "Ogino singlehandedly put natural family planning on a solid scientific basis."

Still, natural family planning had a long way to go.

Before proceeding, let us look at female fertility. A woman becomes fertile when, and only when, she ovulates. Ovulation is the release of an egg. If not fertilized, the egg dies within twelve to twenty-four hours. This means that, strictly speaking, a woman is fertile for no more than twenty-four hours each cycle.

However, the male sperm can survive in her body for up to four days. So intercourse during a stretch of about five days can produce a child, since sperm can be awaiting the egg for 4 days, or be received on the very day the egg is released.

Others read the evidence differently, saying that a rare second ovulation, as in the case of fraternal twins, can occur within twenty-four hours of the first ovulation. This would extend the possible time of fertilization to forty-eight hours. They say that sperm can survive for about five days. Those who use these figures hold that intercourse during a period of about seven days can produce a child. (Multiple ovulations are more likely in women who are taking fertility drugs, as NFP teachers should inform learners.)

If a woman could know ahead of time the very *minute* she was to ovulate in this cycle, NFP would be delightfully simple: to have a child, have intercourse within hours of ovulation; to exclude conception, abstain from four days before to one day after ovulation.

This is where Ogino came partly to the rescue with calendar rhythm. He could not pinpoint ovulation, but he could and did say that it would normally occur between the twelfth and sixteenth day before the next menstruation. The theory was that by keeping a record of her past cycles, she could rely on them to say, "The present cycle will be no longer than the longest past cycle, and no shorter than the shortest past cycle." On this basis, by simple calculation, she could pinpoint the days within which the fertile period would occur. (The formula was: the shortest cycle minus nineteen days equals the start of possible fertility; the longest cycle minus ten days equals the start of post-ovulatory infertility.)

Let us review the limitations of calendar rhythm. First, the only input from the woman's body was the length of her *past* cycles. Second, she made no other self-observations. Third, she knew only by hindsight when ovulation took place. When menstruation began, she could say, "I ovulated twelve to sixteen days ago." The system was built on the hope, not always rewarded, that her body would follow the norm pre-set in her earlier cycles. That was the major limitation of the old rhythm method.

The next advance was the Basal Body Temperature Method (BBT). It capitalized on the long-known fact that when an egg is released, the "yellow body" which contained it begins to release progesterone. This hormone both inhibits further ovulation and triggers a body temperature rise.

With BBT, the woman takes her temperature each morning on awakening and records it. When the rising temperature pattern fits the one she had learned, she concludes that the fertile period has passed, so that there is no likelihood of conception before the next menstruation and subsequent ovulation.

Notice the advance. The woman has passed from theory to self observation. Her own body is telling her of her fertility pattern. True, she only knows that ovulation has occurred *after* it happens each time, but this is enough solid information to assure her that she cannot presently conceive. This method is highly effective for determining post-ovulation infertility. Its drawback is that it restricts intercourse to the period between the temperature rise and the next menstruation.

A German researcher, Dr. G. K. Doring, began to use the temperature curve from previous cycles to calculate very accurately the end of pre-ovulation infertility. However, the more common system used in the late 1940's was a combination of a calendar rule for pre-ovulation infertility and the temperature for post-ovulation infertility.

Next came a development which the users of the ovulation method consider one of the most significant in the history of NFP. It had been observed as far back as 1855 that cervical mucus increased at a certain time in the woman's cycle. By 1932, Latz and Reiner had come to recognize that this increase of mucus could be used to signal the approach of ovulation.

In 1937, J. G. H. Holt had written: "Ovulation, whether or not accompanied by the characteristic pain, is usually attended by one or more outward signs. Almost always a slight mucus discharge is perceptible for some days round about the time of ovulation. I am of the opinion that this symptom will occur in all healthy women."

In 1949, Dr. Edward Keefe, a New York gynecologist, included a note on this symptom in the first handbook with his specially sensitive *Ovulindex* thermometer for use with the temperature method. He recommended keeping "careful record" of the "clear vaginal discharge" seen for a few days before ovulation, to help tell the time of fertility.

But it was not until the 1950's that the significance of this symptom began to be stressed as a help to users of NFP. By 1953, Dr. Keefe was describing the characteristics of the mucus, and encouraging his patients to observe it at the vulva (the opening of the vagina) as a sign of approaching ovulation, as was taught by Holt.

His patients soon observed a new sign: the cervix tended to open and rise at the time of greatest fertility. By 1962, Dr. Keefe had entered this information into the medical literature.

In 1953, Drs. John and Evelyn Billings began to single out the mucus sign and devote painstaking research to its nature. Dr. Josef Roetzer was also using the mucus symptom in Europe. Dr. Hanna Klaus writes, "The credit for the painstaking recording of the initial mucus observation, together with correlation of mucus and the cyclic hormones, is due to the Billings, James Brown and Henry Burger." Dr. Billings first fielded a mucus-temperature system of NFP. By 1964 he had written the first edition of *The Ovulation Method.* By 1971 he was teaching that the mucus could be observed at the vulva and used by itself as a basis for natural family planning. Its appearance is a positive sign that the fertile time is present. Its disappearance for a certain number of days is a sign of post-ovulatory infertility.

What happens is that before ovulation the cervix produces a copious, wet, stretchy mucus. When it flows down the vagina, it appears at the vulva. Many women can feel it at the vulva. A woman can confirm its presence by a tissue paper examination. NFP instructors teach a woman the details of using the sign to know when she is fertile and when not. The mucus symptom can be used by itself as the ovulation method (OM). It can also be used as part of the sympto-thermal method, which combines the mucus symptom with the temperature observation, and sometimes with other symptoms.

The medical explanation of the mucus flow is illuminating, and confirms its meaning as a sign of fertility. Generally, the vagina is dry and non-supportive of sperm. Any mucus present is so structured that it acts like a roadblock to entering sperm. Soon after the ovulation process starts, the cervical mucus discharge begins, frequently as a rather tacky or sticky substance. As the woman gets closer to ovulation, it becomes wet and stretchy as a result of the release of the hormone estrogen. This wet mucus helps the sperm along on its journey to fertilize the egg.

Awareness of these developments in gynecological knowledge is perhaps the surest way to cure the stubborn and almost obsessive distrust of natural methods which still prevails. Most women already know of the mucus changes but have no idea of the treasury of family planning information they contain.

Besides these developments, we have a new awareness of nature's old, unassisted method of child spacing: breast-feeding. Common in third world countries, it has spread rapidly in the U.S. because of women's growing awareness of its benefits for the baby.

Breast-feeding tends to suppress ovulation, thus providing a period of infertility. This is not to say that untutored breast-feeding is as reliable as modern methods of birth control. Still, until modern times, when millions of women discontinued breast-feeding, it served as a moderating influence on family size and population growth. In many countries it still does.

There is now a carefully tutored form of breast-feeding more scientifically related to ovulation suppression. It is called "ecological breast-feeding." In one study by the Couple to Couple League, mothers using this form of breast-feeding averaged 14.6 months without any menstrual periods or menstrual bleeding. The Couple to Couple League (CCL) may be unique in its advocacy of ecological breast-feeding. Interested mothers should contact CCL and read Sheila Kippley's book, *Breast-feeding and Natural Child Spacing*.

4. Has the Ovulation Method made the Temperature Method obsolete, along with calendar rhythm?

You might say that the Ovulation Method has given the Basal Body Temperature Method (BBT) a higher life. BBT is now used in combination with the mucus symptom. Together they are called the Sympto-Thermal Method. Thus the two modern methods are the Ovulation Method (OM) and the Sympto-Thermal Method.

OM is a method complete in itself. The Family of the Americas, which provides the Billings Method, offers only OM. Dr. Billings insists that OM is reliable, simple and all that is needed. Many others, from researchers to practiced teachers, feel the same.

The Sympto-Thermal Method (STM) combines mucus and temperature as a double-check method. It also employs other symptoms such as the changing condition of the cervix.

The cervix signals approaching ovulation by softening and dilating; it signals the passing of ovulation by closing and becoming firm again.

Advocates of STM stress the added security given by these cross-checks. They also point out that when one or other symptom is doubtful, the others fill in for it. They declare that the mere disappearance of the mucus does not provide the positive assurance that ovulation has taken place, but the temperature rise does. Ovulation may fail to occur with the first appearance of mucus and may occur in a second appearance. In this case, the absence of ovulation is indicated by the lack of a temperature rise after the first mucus occurrence.

Of course, temperature rise can originate from causes such as the common cold or other illnesses. NFP instructors teach users the due cautions in using temperature for NFP.

A woman with inadequate mucus may find temperature or cervix a better sign than mucus that the post-ovulatory infertile phase has begun.

It is for these reasons that many NFP professionals, both researchers and teachers, prefer to teach and promote STM.

Which method is better? I cannot settle that question. Statistics to be given later confirm the validity of both methods. One method has certain advantages, and the other has other advantages. Which better fits a couple's needs and preferences?

Teachers will teach the method they are convinced is better, but should be ready to help a couple who may prefer another method. A couple should learn all the symptoms, and decide whether to use OM or STM, or the Temperature Method alone.

John Kippley, co-founder of the Couple to Couple League, told me, "I know from personal correspondence and informal surveys that some people who have taken STM instruction from CCL use a mucus-only system, and others use a temperature-only system. Probably most use mucus and temperature as a cross-check. I don't care which method they choose, but I feel very strongly about teaching them all the signs and how they can be used as a cross-check. Thus we give them the freedom to choose based on their own personal experience."

5. Is NFP hard to learn?

The World Health Organization (WHO) set out to research the answer to this question as it concerns the Ovulation Method. It commissioned a five-country study of OM with a follow-up analysis. Eight hundred and sixty-nine women, from illiterates to college grads and beyond, were chosen from both rural and urban populations.

In the very first cycle, 93% recorded an interpretable ovulatory mucus pattern, and 90% had a good-to-excellent grasp of the method.

This is more impressive since these women were not shown mucus pattern charts (as is normal in training), for fear they might imitate instead of observe, and ruin the results. They were simply told that each woman has her own pattern, and must observe it. And they did.

The WHO study provides an authoritative answer to our question. Given qualified teachers, most women readily learn OM. However, the learning process should go on. Women have to learn to deal with irregular cycles and the complications of post-partum, breast-feeding and menopause. NFP can handle them all, but the couple must learn to handle NFP.

Both OM and STM are commonly taught to couples in one to four sessions of about two hours each. Typically, books for further study and charts for recording observations (plus a thermometer in the case of STM) are distributed at the first session. Teachers may make themselves available by phone for problem cases. One important objective is that couples learn together.

At the second session, teachers review the couples' charts, make suggestions and/or corrections, and go deeper into methods. The basics of NFP are easy to learn. Women with complicated cycles or scant symptoms have more of a problem. Absence of expected symptoms can point to a health problem. If it is resolved, the expected symptoms generally appear.

Through NFP training and use, some couples discover that their fertility is low. Many couples are just not very fertile, and would have no more than two or three children without any family planning. In the United States, about one couple in six is infertile.

A woman with scant symptoms because of her low fertility can have difficulty with NFP. She is planning to avoid what is not likely to happen in any case, and nature is withholding the usual signs. Her NFP teachers may be able to help her solve the problem, either directly or by referral to the medical consultant nearly every program has.

Through NFP, low fertility couples learn how to maximize the possibility of conception. NFP has brought many couples the joy of having a child without recourse to expensive treatment.

For most couples, the learning process is not too demanding. However, by continuing to learn more, a couple can gain added confidence, avoid mistakes and even reduce the days of necessary abstinence.

6. Should NFP be learned before or after marriage?

This question has vexed many teachers for fear that unmarried teens will misuse what they learn. However, girls have a right to know their own bodies. Furthermore, Dr. Hanna Klaus, who has taught fertility awareness to girls, has found that it helps to develop in them an appreciation and reverence for their fertility and a greater responsibility for it. In her pilot group of 235, the girls readily learned to distinguish when they ovulated and when they did not. Half of the sub-group which had initiated sexual activity before they entered the program discontinued the practice.

In his great document *Familiaris Consortio* (Role Of The Christian Family In the Modern World), Pope John Paul II has expressly stated that fertility awareness should be taught before marriage. He wrote that "every effort must be made to render such knowledge accessible to all married people, and also to young adults before marriage, through clear, timely and serious instruction and education given by married couples, doctors and experts" (n. 33).

Fr. Marc Caligari, S.J., who taught at Brophy College Prep, Phoenix, integrated fertility awareness into his marriage and chastity course for high school students. He was able not only to teach all the Catholic religious and moral values attached to sexuality, but also to show how they can be lived.

Some priests have required engaged couples to take instruction in NFP before setting their wedding date. The results in one diocese were that every single couple afterward expressed gratitude for what they had learned about themselves, even though some were initially opposed. Many, but not all, used the method. Their experience eloquently attests that far too little has been done of what can and must be done by bishops, priests, doctors and religious educators to see that couples are instructed in the one method of family planning that makes it possible for them to keep the moral law without heroic sacrifice.

The gynecologist, Dr. Charles W. Norris, who is passionately convinced of the value of NFP, has co-authored *Know Your Body*. This book integrates NFP into a family-oriented treatment of human sexuality and is invaluable for sex education courses.

7. If NFP is that good, why haven't I heard more about it? How many people use it?

The question supposes that any truly worthwhile development is quickly trumpeted abroad in our media-saturated culture. Unhappily, this is not true. Why not? In the case of NFP, we can consider three major reasons: little felt need for NFP; inadequate leadership; and media non-cooperation.

Until the last five to ten years, many people thought that contraceptive technology had solved the problem of family planning, despite the Church's opposition. So there was little felt need for a new method. That meant NFP did not qualify as news.

However, the medical drawbacks of contraceptives grew more serious and became better known. At the same time, the family and social deterioration caused by the sexual revolution continued to escalate. Prodded by the insistent teaching of Popes Paul VI and John Paul II, at least some people began to rethink their attitude toward contraception. One graduate student said, "Wouldn't it be awful if the Pope had approved of the pill? Now they'd be blaming the Church for all these side effects. And there would be no NFP." At any rate, in a September, 1985 survey by *U.S. Catholic*, 30% of the respondents stated that using artificial means of birth control is sinful.

The second reason for the slow spread of NFP is inadequate leadership. A small number of doctors, priests, religious and lay people led the way in NFP, but the majority have still not become involved.

Priests: NFP teachers and users anguish over the lack of support from priests. Once when I referred to NFP in a homily, a NFP teacher thanked me and said it was the first time in several years that she had heard it mentioned from the pulpit. I once asked a priest friend who had preached against contraception why he never mentioned NFP. He stated, "I know nothing about it." This is the state of affairs. Busy priests are hard-pressed to keep up with developments in a changing Church—but NFP is one development they can't afford to neglect. I agree with John Kippley of the Couple to Couple League that preaching against contraception should never be done without also referring to the NFP solution.

Doctors: The lack of support from doctors also troubles NFP teachers and practitioners. The reasons for this are even more complex than that for the lack of priestly leadership in the issue, even though NFP is more in the doctors' domain than the priests'. An article in the winter, 1985 issue of the *International Review of Natural Family Planning* probes one significant reason for this lack: medical journals. "Journals of obstetrics and gynecology and reproductive medicine," the authors observe, "play a major role in the formation of a physician's practice."

The authors of the article did a study of the advertisements in five journals of obstetrics and gynecology. They learned that the five journals earned a minimum of $1,751,097 (26% of advertising revenues) for ads "aimed at abating or destroying fertility." These ads are *informative*. They provide busy physicians with a continuous contraceptive update. Where can physicians get a similar time-saving update on NFP?

Because NFP is non-profit, its promoters cannot finance

expensive ads on its behalf. And ads are not the whole story. Dr. Hanna Klaus reports that "it took several years and at least two personal visits to every physician in the U.S. by 'drug detail' men" before birth control pills began to have a sizeable market. NFP supporters have not, and perhaps cannot, mount such efforts. Doctors are often too busy to ferret it out for themselves from the disinformation served by the media. If individuals supplied the best available literature to doctors, it would bear fruit.

These reasons begin to explain why NFP is not better known. A look at the media tells more of the story.

The media elite: A survey reported in the *Washington Post*, and reprinted in the newsletter of the Catholic League for Religious and Civil Rights, revealed some astonishing facts. 50% of the media elite have no religious affiliation. 86% seldom or never attend religious services. 54% do not regard adultery as wrong, and almost universally they stand opposed to sexual constraints by either government or tradition. Knowing this, it's understandable that the media has not given favorable coverage to NFP.

The media is more than a roadblock to NFP. It is a counterforce. It misinforms. It has yet to accept even the title "Natural Family Planning." Instead, it almost always refers to NFP as "the rhythm method," if it even mentions it at all. As this writer wrote to one of the most prestigious papers in the country, such labeling only perpetuates an error. We in NFP expect from such prestigious papers "the same learned reflection of developments and changing terminology which it gives to others," rather than this "aggravating impediment" to all working in the NFP field.

An Associated Press article by Joan Mower (8/27/85) seven times equated NFP with the rhythm method, and termed NFP "a cruel hoax." As the writer pointed out to the newspaper which published the article locally, "The hoax is to talk about rhythm at all. No one is teaching it." *Psychology Today* (June, 1983), spoke of NFP as "Rhythm Revisited," and left the impression that consistent cycle regularity is necessary. Would you recognize NFP in this distortion?

I have yet to see a newspaper article honestly report the favorable studies of NPF's effectiveness. One newspaper columnist wrote derogatorily that NFP is "an updated version of rhythm," (which, left unexplained, is misleading), and "one of the least effective methods of preventing pregnancy"—which is false. She proceeded to "prove" it by stating that "a World Health Organization Study showed that 35% of the women who use the method in the third world give up after 13 months. Half of them give it up because they are pregnant." Here are the facts she didn't report: of the 35 per hundred who "give up" the method, 19.6 had become pregnant (of which only 2.8 were method failures), 6.6 quit (temporarily?) to become pregnant, 5.2 had moved away, 3.6 had separated from spouses, etc. Only six per hundred left the method because of dissatisfaction. This is an extremely low rate of dissatisfaction and dropout for any method. Even 35% is low, as she should have informed her readers. Why did she not? I can only report that the article was an attack on government policy, which is finally providing some significant funding specifically for NFP. The writer complained, "Supporters of natural family planning argue that the method isn't at fault, people are. But how do you call the method a success if the patient is pregnant?" The fact is that these were women of proven fertility with a mean average age of 30.1 years, and over 45% had said they planned to have more children, but not immediately. Apparently, some changed their minds, to the displeasure of the columnist.

As Dr. Hanna Klaus has stated, "When you really get down to looking at what is implied and imagined—absolute need for contraception—what one is really saying is that the sexual drive is outside the control of a person, that people don't have free will. Where does that leave them? In an effort to try to make life better for them, one is really denying that which gives us dignity as human beings: our freedom."

Despite these obstacles, NFP is spreading. It is difficult to obtain figures. Polls are expensive. In a 1982 review of all aspects of NFP, researcher-teacher Dr. Hanna Klaus gave a few statistics. NFP users in the U.S. stood at 2.8% in 1973, and rose to 3.4% in 1976. This amounted to one and one-half million couples. In 1980, over 100,000 couples trained in NFP.

In 1982, Larry Kane of the Human Life and Natural Family Planning Foundation reported that diocesan-related NFP sites grew from 42 in 1970 to more than 1,000 by 1982.

On the government level, both the U.S. and the U.N. have become active in NFP. The Department of Health and Human Services requires that funded centers of family planning teach NFP or give referrals. It is also providing curricula for teaching doctors, nurses, and the public. By 1986, the U.S. Agency for International Development had "dramatically increased its spending" on outlays for NFP.

A 1983 survey showed that a third of U.S. Catholic hospitals had begun NFP programs, and over half of the others were interested.

Many foreign countries have NFP programs, including at least eleven in the Americas.

With most people reluctant to speak about an intimate subject like their method of family planning, and with the media's negativity and neglect, the word about NFP spreads slowly. That is why you have not heard more about it.

But you will. NFP has arrived. Dr. Klaus reported that it is the fastest growing reversible method of family planning.

8. How effective is NFP?

Its effectiveness is rated at 97% to 99%. This means that if one hundred women learned and used the method perfectly for a year, only one to three of those women would have an unplanned pregnancy. This is as effective as the mini-pill, and is better than the IUD, diaphragm and condom.

In practice, not all learn the method perfectly and, as with every method, not all use it faithfully. Therefore we talk about *use effectiveness* as well as *method effectiveness*.

"Use effectiveness" expresses the results measured in actual use. Because couples who use the method are not as reliable as the method, use effectiveness of NFP is generally lower than the 97-99% method effectiveness reported above.

Since use effectiveness depends on the reliability of the users, different surveys show divergent results. Rather than start with the most favorable results, we will look at a study done by a well-known sponsor: the World Health Organization study of the Ovulation Method (referred to in the answer to question five) entitled: *A Prospective Multicentre Trial of the Ovulation Method of Natural Family Planning. II. The Effectiveness Phase.*

The results of the entire five-country study among women using the method to avoid a pregnancy were as follows: rated in terms of one hundred women using OM for a year, the pregnancy rate was 22.3%. That is, 22.3 women out of a hundred were pregnant.

That sounds very high, but consider the rest of the data: of the 22.3 pregnancies per one hundred women, 15.4 were traced to what is called *informed choice pregnancies*. In addition, 3.9 were discovered to be from inaccurate application of instructions (the couples either did not learn correctly or did not correctly use what they learned); another 0.3 pregnancies per hundred were shown to have resulted from *faulty teaching*; and a study of the couples' reports and charts indicated that 2.2 pregnancies per hundred couples were method related (that is, these couples kept to the rules, but became pregnant). Finally, there was no evident cause why 0.5 pregnancies per hundred occurred. They may have resulted from any of the above causes, but could not be traced.

Now let's see what these data tell us. First, look at the informed choice pregnancies. *Informed choice* means that during the study, some couples changed their minds and decided to become pregnant, and others knowingly departed from the rules, hoping not to become pregnant, but did. (Good teachers warn couples that "taking chances" is really "planning a pregnancy.")

If we subtract from the 22.3 pregnant women these 15.4 *informed choice* pregnancies, we are left with only 6.9 women out of a hundred who kept to the rules but became pregnant in a year.

What if we also subtract the pregnancies resulting from imperfect teaching (0.3), and from imperfect learning or use (3.9)? We do this on the supposition that these imperfections can be eliminated. We find that we are now down to 2.7 pregnancies per hundred women per year.

Further, if we assume that the 0.5 uncertain-cause pregnancies may also have resulted from failure to teach or learn correctly, we subtract the 0.5 from the 2.7, and have only 2.2 pregnancies among one hundred women in a year. This figure agrees with the number of method-related failures actually tabulated by study of the conduct and charts of the participants.

The fact that the source of only 0.5% of the pregnancies in the study could not be pinned down points out the scientific nature of NFP.

How effective NFP proves to be depends primarily on how well it is taught, and how motivated couples are not to have a child at present. The World Health Organization study makes this clear.

Where poverty and population pressures are high, as in India, people are showing how reliable NFP is. Dr. Sr. Catherine Bernard reports on a 1984 prospective study of almost ten thousand couples. The pregnancy rate was less than two per hundred women per year, including all causes, such as deliberate departure from the method, which is called "informed choice pregnancy."

Where there is grave reason to avoid pregnancy, NFP comes through in a unique way. It is the only method with a sliding scale of effectiveness adjustable to need. Austrian Dr. Josef Roetzer, of world renown in NFP, treats of this sliding scale in his book *Family Planning the Natural Way*. He gives directions for using the Sympto-Thermal Method where "pregnancy avoidance is a matter of life or death." This highest-effective use of NFP requires additional abstinence. It is based on the medical fact that, when the post-ovulatory phase of the cycle is properly identified, there is almost no possibility that intercourse can produce a pregnancy.

In the September 18, 1993 issue of the prestigious *British Medical Journal*, R. E. J. Ryder, M.D., reviews the various NFP reliability studies. He sums up by saying that "the accumulating data confirm that natural family planning can be as effective as any method of family planning."

Hardship cases do exist. Some women with sparse mucus and irregular cycles may find they cannot use the Ovulation Method, but can use the Sympto-Thermal Method with its multiple indicators. Others may have to be referred to a nutritionist, or to the medical consultant of the training program they attend.

NFP is effective in another way. At the second session of a two-session training program the author attended, one couple did not return. After the first session, they achieved the pregnancy they had been attempting for two years.

The Feminists for Life of Columbus, Ohio, issued a paper on the Ovulation Method which states: "The only disadvantage I can find to it is that you cannot get pregnant 'accidentally' any more. You know when you are fertile, even when you don't want to know." That statement is very close to the truth about the effectiveness of NFP. Except for a marginal upper limit, it is almost as effective as a couple cares to make it.

9. Everything has its disadvantages. What are the disadvantages of NFP? How many days of abstinence are required?

Among the disadvantages of NFP, it lacks the automatic results of the pill, the IUD and sterilization. It does not allow one spouse to pile on the other the sacrifices involved in family planning. It requires that the couple learn the method. They must respect their fertility and use their intelligence, monitor their fertility indicators, record the cycles, and achieve the self-mastery necessary to meet their family planning obligations. In summary, it requires them to live in harmony with nature and one another, and not take an escape route from either.

These could be labeled as disadvantages. But more accurately they are *costs*, the cost of investing in the very best in family planning. Every way of life has its costs, and NFP is a way of life.

One cost of every family planning method is the possibility of failure. Here, couples who have embraced NFP have a distinct advantage. They have accepted responsibility for their power of fertility. They keep it in their hands, integrate it into the rhythms of their marital relationship, and entrust the weight of it to their free wills. As a result, they are better disposed to be accepting if they do not live up to their plans. If they are a religious couple, they know that God acts through their procreative powers. Should there be what we call a "method failure," they accept it as his part in their family planning. Thus, in either method failure or user failure, they know that God calls them to accept and love the child they had not planned. Many couples have proved their responsibility and nobility by welcoming an unplanned pregnancy, which gives them a much-loved child.

If the spouses are not mature and loving enough to readily achieve this wholesome respect for each other's body and nature, they face hardships until they mature. NFP requires growth, and growth involves sacrifice, a going out from where we are to arrive at what we want to be and can become.

NFP requires an honest exchange of concerns, and airing of feelings. It calls for patience and humor. At one training session, a wife asked how she could remain in bed in the morning for even the few minutes required to take her temperature if she awoke to the children crying. The instructor explained, "Your husband can get up." The husband retorted, "*She* can get up. I'll take *my* temperature!" All present burst into laughter, as the husband had intended.

Times of disturbed cycles, postpartum, and menopause can cause anxiety and can lengthen the required abstinence.

Some mature couples who are not religious bear with these costs for reasons that have nothing to do with faith, except their faith in one another. They shame Christians who reject the cross and who, if they will use it, have the advantage of the example of Christ. He paid the cost of his bond with his spouse the Church without considering it a disadvantage. Love doesn't heed such costs.

Another possible cost of NFP hinges around a question: does a woman's sexual desire peak at the very time abstinence is called for? No doubt some women's desire peaks together with the fertile period. One could argue that it should for all, since nature is set on producing children. But research says no. "Almost every phase of the cycle," writes Nona Aguilar, "has been shown to coincide with peak desire for at least some women."

If peak desire and ovulation coincided, no other NFP symptoms would be needed! Women would *know* when they are fertile.

Some women claim that the two do peak together, but they may simply be experiencing the effect of abstinence. It is the best aphrodisiac. But no doubt there are women whose sexual desire peaks at abstinence time. For them, this is a special cost of NFP. One can only suggest that love is better than sex, and love at all times is better than sex on demand. Woman after woman reports a deepening of spousal tenderness and love through NFP. It makes sense. Abstinence is an aphrodisiac for the husband too.

When the abstinence period has passed, a husband who loves his wife will elicit her longing with his love. Expressions of love are more powerful in awakening amatory desires than the cycles of nature.

The number of days of abstinence required to practice NFP vary so much between couples, and even with the same couple, that teachers are reluctant to quote figures. Yet the question can certainly be answered statistically.

The author invited Dr. Hanna Klaus to discuss this question with Mr. Jeff Spieler, who was involved in the cited five-country WHO study of OM. Mr. Spieler said that after the learning period, abstinence averaged 15.4 days in a 28.6 day cycle. This figure includes both the period of menstruation, and the alternate days of abstinence recommended during the pre-ovulatory period. The 13.2 days left for non-fertile intercourse each cycle occur in part before ovulation, and in part after. The longest period of abstinence at a stretch averaged 9.5 days.

Dr. Klaus replied that *practiced* users of OM don't require the pre-ovulatory alternate days of abstinence; thus, for them, abstinence would be somewhat less. She also noted that the number of days available easily accommodates the intercourse frequency of many couples who do not use NFP. Therefore, what NFP shifts is not the frequency of intercourse but its pattern.

On another occasion when the writer consulted Dr. Klaus, she was even more specific. She stated that the average length of necessary abstinence for the Ovulation Method is 8.5 days plus/minus three days for each cycle. This excludes the days of menstruation, which some avoid anyway for other reasons, but which NFP beginners *must* avoid until the woman can distinguish the mucus symptom from the menstrual flow.

The Sympto-Thermal Method makes comparable abstinence requirements, but it does not require abstinence during the menses except for the first two learning cycles.

10. Who is ready for all those days of abstinence?

The millions who are using NPF can accept some days of abstinence, as well as the uncounted millions more who would, if only someone would usher them into its secrets. The question of difficulty is meaningless without relating it to the motivation stirred by the values gained.

Motivation can't always be chopped into categories and put in words. There are reasons of the mind and reasons of the heart. But let us consider the motives which people report and the motives which are evident.

In the WHO study referred to earlier, 40.6% adopted NFP for religious reasons; 23.8% because they were dissatisfied, or anticipated dissatisfaction, with other methods; 3.2% because they couldn't use other methods; and 16.4% for reasons not tabulated.

All of these reasons spell human drama and the stories of human hearts. Some couples pay the cost of abstinence because they are committed to obeying the teaching Church; some to live in tune with their bodies; some because their bodies cannot tolerate contraceptives, or have been harmed by them; some because they're frightened by the medical reports on contraceptives; some because their spouses are tired of bearing all the costs of family planning; some because the "freedom" of contraceptives was too demanding on their sexual nature; some because they learned their contraceptive was an abortifacient; and some because they abhor sterilization. Some were dragooned into taking an NFP course, and were delighted by what they learned. Others came because of low fertility. They practice abstinence during the infertile time to gather their fullest powers of life-giving for the fertile time in the hope of having a child.

These, and others who have ventured into NFP and learned its rewards, often tell their own stories in touching ways. For a deep look into the lives and psychology of some of them, read Nona Aguilar's *New No-Pill, No-Risk Birth Control,* or Mary Shivanandan's *Challenge To Love.* The latter book also discusses the spiritual experiences fostered by NFP.

For a veteran teacher's excellent treatment of the *why* of NFP, from ecology, effectiveness and low cost, through health, moral and religious reasons—and the rest of the story and practice of NFP as well—see *The Art Of Natural Family Planning* by John. F. Kippley, co-founder of the Couple To Couple League.

Abstinence can challenge a couple, but love meets the challenge. Many who have made the sacrifice have found the hardships shrinking as they enter a new land rich in promises to be explored.

Except for sterilization, many contraceptives are losing adherents, even though experimental new ones like injectable contraceptives are coming along and enticing users. Though poor in numbers, NFP may still be one of the fastest growing methods. People want its rewards. They are taking on its challenge of abstinence.

11. Where does that leave people who like to do everything spontaneously? Can NFP accommodate such free spirits?

Let us begin by reflecting on life itself. It accommodates all types, but not always. Impulsiveness and spontaneity have their seasons; discipline does too. No one can be both fully mature and fully spontaneous. Infants are the only fully spontaneous humans. For both moral and social reasons, and for the sake of reason itself, human maturation involves learning to moderate impulses, whims and tendencies.

In *Neurotic Styles,* a clinical study of neurosis, Dr. David Shapiro writes, "In many respects the psychopath is the very model of the impulsive style."

Each of us has two sets of drives: one to spontaneity, the other to self control. Simple survival requires the moderating of spontaneity; successful living requires its happy blending with self control.

Is NFP compatible with a moderately spontaneous lifestyle? Of course. Some successfully harmonize a moderately spontaneous lifestyle with complete premarital chastity and with monogamous marriage and natural family planning.

The channeling of primitive energies into nobler goals is called sublimation. Successful marriage requires generous levels of sublimation. Couples separated for a time by reason of occupation or the call to serve their country, or simply by protracted illness, have through the centuries expressed their loving faithfulness by abstinence.

When planning a child, NFP couples have months and years of full spontaneity in joyous intercourse that is harmonized with all the qualities of conscience and virtue. That is true marital and sexual bliss.

If sound and serious reasons counsel spacing or limiting children, they have days and weeks when they put a reign on their impulsiveness for a noble cause. They sublimate their sexual energies into the same tender kisses and embraces by which chaste premarital couples have always expressed their affection. These varieties of love improve their marital relationship.

The fact is that few things drain the thrill from marital sex faster than unvarying total availability. Women's journals bear witness to the boredom that sex joined to contraception has spawned. NFP couples express a contrary experience. They may experience some problems, but not dullness. You are more likely to hear them describe their life together as alternating periods of courtship and honeymoon.

Couples who practice the periodic spontaneity that is in keeping with God's law will reap the rewards of marital joy and peace.

12. Would you explain further why NFP is morally and religiously acceptable?

Catholicism and some other religions accept only two types of conduct for fertility control: abstinence for the unmarried, and periodic abstinence among the married who have serious reason to space or limit children.

NFP is acceptable because it allows the married couple to give themselves to one another completely and totally in each marital act, in accord with their marriage covenant. It is the ideal religious, moral and ecological method. The couple practice it in their purely natural state, using nothing but their intelligence, self-knowledge, self-observation and self-controlled timing of intercourse.

Because of its wholesome, non-invasive character, NFP is spreading among Christians, Moslems, Hindus, Buddhists and others. Some five percent of teachers and medical professionals in China use NFP.

The Catholic Church, alert and compassionate to the need for morally acceptable family planning, was a prime mover in the development of modern NFP.

With the bishops of the world assembled, the Second Vatican Council stated that medical, biological and other scientists "can considerably advance the welfare of marriage and the family, along with peace of conscience if by pooling their efforts they labor to explain more thoroughly the various conditions favoring a proper regulation of births" (*Gaudium et Spes,* n. 52).

Pope Paul VI, who dealt so wrenchingly with the issue of family planning, referred to this text in his encyclical *On The Regulation Of Births (Humanae Vitae)*. He also referred to Pope Pius XII who, in 1951, encouraged medical science to look for a secure natural way of birth regulation. Then he added his voice to the appeal.

Now that NFP has been developed so successfully, Pope John Paul II never tires of recommending it. He explains why in his document *Familiaris Consortio*. He marvels at how "the experience of many couples" and the data of science attest to the profound advantages of NFP. Not least of these is the fact that "The choice of the natural rhythms involves accepting the cycle of the person, that is the woman, and thereby accepting dialogue, reciprocal respect, shared responsibility and self-control" (n. 32).

Morally and religiously, NFP is not simply grudgingly accepted by the Church. It has been brought into being in part by the passionate appeals of compassionate churchmen. It is praised and propagated as the answer of God and nature and researchers to the crying modern need for a holy, healthy, reliable method of family planning.

NFP is morally and religiously acceptable because it is a good means to a good end: family planning.

13. Since NFP has the same purpose as contraception, why isn't the one method as morally acceptable as the other?

Actually, they don't have the same purpose. The purpose of contraceptives is to suppress fertility. The purpose of NFP is to guide conduct so a couple can live wisely with their unsuppressed fertility. Let us look at the issues involved.

To act morally is to act in harmony with our nature as we know it by reason. To act religiously is to act in harmony with both reason and revelation. Catholic morality is based on reason and revelation as authoritatively interpreted by the Church.

Before we can say whether an act is good or bad, both its means and its end must be judged. Take a simple example: one man buys a car and another man steals one. The act of the first man is moral because he used a good means to the end. The act of the second man is immoral because he used a bad means to *the same end*.

The end does not justify the means. Both must be good.

To attain its good end of family planning, NFP uses only the good means of intelligence, observation and self control. By using these good means, it acts in perfect harmony with human nature to attain its end.

The end of contraceptive behavior is to suppress fertility by invading the body or perverting the act of intercourse itself. It is a bad end and therefore immoral.

Those who use contraceptives or contraceptive behavior intend fertility suppression for the sake of family planning. This is wrong because it is not in harmony with human nature. They attack a part of themselves to get what they want. They are doing something wrong to gain something right. That is immoral. Both the means and the end must be good before an act is moral. Therefore contraceptive family planning is immoral.

Contraceptive family planning is immoral whether it uses suppressive drugs and devices, contraceptive sterilization or contraceptive behavior. Contraceptive behavior includes any action that sets out to produce orgasm in an abnormal way.

In the broadest sense, all have the same end of family planning, but only users of NFP employ a means that is moral.

We can approach these same truths in another way. Reason itself sees that the human body has a definite nature, and organs with definite purposes. For instance, the nature of the eye is to see. People don't put out their eyes when they want to sleep. They try to find a dark place.

Nature attracts man and woman to one another in the stable sexual union of marriage. Sexual union is by nature both an act of love and an act open to new life. Repressing either love or the possibility of life-giving is wrong. A man who virtually rapes his wife—having no regard for her feelings or her conscience, and threatening her for refusal to comply—commits an immoral act. A man who loves a woman but suppresses his fertility by contraception because he doesn't want a child also commits an immoral act.

Interference with fertility warps the nature of a couple's sexual union and cheats on their total mutual self-giving. It is an offense against themselves, their marriage covenant, and their God who made them share in his creativity. The Church insists on these truths.

Pope John Paul II gives a summary of this doctrine in a passage of *Familiaris Consortio*: "When couples, by means of recourse to contraception, separate these two meanings (of mutual self-giving and human procreation) that God the Creator has inscribed in the being of man and woman in the dynamism of their sexual communion, they act as 'arbiters' of the divine plan and they 'manipulate' and degrade human sexuality—and with it themselves and their married partner—by altering its value of 'total' self-giving. Thus the innate language that expresses the total reciprocal self-giving of husband and wife is overlaid, through contraception, by an objectively contradictory language, namely, that of not giving oneself totally to the other. This leads not only to a positive refusal to be open to life but also to a falsification of the inner truth of conjugal love, which is called upon to give itself in personal totality" (n. 32).

In this light, one can see it is no accident that many women feel "used" when year after year they use contraceptives to supply their husbands with sex-without-responsibility. And men who render themselves sterile are equally used. And always, both are degraded.

Books have been written on this subject, such as John Kippley's *Sex And The Marriage Covenant*. He develops the idea that, in God's plan, the marital act always, at least implicitly, renews the faith and caring love that the couple pledged one another when they married. It is meant to be a renewal of their marriage covenant.

Persons who take a cue about rightness and wrongness from manifestly holy people should know that Padre Pio, the priest who had the five wounds of Christ mystically, opposed contraception. He used to assure people that God would forgive them if they repented. On September 23, 1968, eleven days before he died, he wrote in a letter to Pope Paul VI: "I thank you for your clear and decisive words that you especially pronounced in the latest encyclical *Humanae Vitae* and I reaffirm my faith and my unconditional obedience to your illuminated directions."

Nobel peace prize winner, Mother Teresa of Calcutta, and her Sisters teach NFP in India. Who could believe that this holy woman, so devoted to the sick and dying, would spend time on any work but the most urgent?

To summarize: all who use family planning may have the same good end, but not all use the only good methods available: fertility awareness and planned abstinence as necessary, or ecological breast-feeding. Contraception attacks human nature. Contraceptive sterilization wounds it permanently.

14. Can NFP be abused?

It can. NFP is good when used for a good purpose, such as avoiding any method that would harm the couple's health. It is good whenever used by a couple to achieve the virtuous purposes of marriage. One of the purposes of marriage is parenthood. Marriage is commitment to a life-long relationship devoted to conjugal love, mutual help, and sexual fulfillment and parenthood. The Second Vatican Council taught, as the Church has always taught, that "marriage and conjugal love are by their nature ordained toward the begetting and educating of children. Children are really the supreme gift of marriage and contribute very substantially to the welfare of their parents" (*Gaudium et Spes*, n. 50).

Human societies have long recognized this. Even in ancient pagan Rome, when the birth rate fell low through abortion and other means, the state stepped in. It required couples who wished to marry to swear before many witnesses that they would bear children.

So NFP is good if used in a good way. This happens when spouses use it to plan and generate their family, in a generous way, in accord with love, reason and faith. It is not only a right but a responsibility of parents to give serious and prayerful consideration to the number of children they can reasonably have and care for. The quote from Pope John Paul II later in this answer will show that. So to use NFP to help in planning a family can be wise, religious, meritorious and praiseworthy.

Of course, if an unplanned child comes along, moral and religious couples will trust in God's providence, and love the child as much as any other. They would never even consider abortion. God forbids it.

Some of the faithful find it hard to accept the idea that there is *any* meritorious way to *plan* a family. They insist couples must rely on divine providence, leaving all planning to God. But St. Thomas Aquinas illumines the matter of divine providence by teaching that part of God's providence is giving us intelligence and a chance to use it. Isn't that what we do in other matters? Why not here? Even before NFP, faithful couples who had grave reason to have no more children planned not having them. They refrained from sexual intercourse.

NFP is an unparalleled help to couples in carrying out virtuous family planning. Use of NFP becomes immoral only when turned to a bad purpose, such as selfishly avoiding the responsibility to bear a family of a size suited to a couple's circumstances.

What about using NFP outside of marriage? Biblical and Church teaching condemn extramarital intercourse; so, too, do many human societies. To use NFP to facilitate premarital sex or adultery is to use it to encourage immorality and sin. Still, those who persist in extramarital intercourse eliminate at least one evil if they use NFP instead of contraception or abortion.

How many children are a couple to bear? That is their decision in the light of all circumstances: religious, personal, social, even national and global. But a few facts can be pointed out. It takes at least 2.1 children per couple to keep a nation's population from decreasing in the long run. In the U.S., as a result of widespread contraception, sterilization and abortion, the average couple is having fewer than that. So even including immigration, there is currently no danger of excessive population growth in the United States, and therefore that is no reason not to have children. Since the population is aging, in the future we will have fewer couples in the childbearing years, so we will need immigration to keep our population from shrinking.

No one should doubt one thing: the Church does *not* teach that a couple should bear as many children as physically possible. Vatican II indicated this, and Pope Paul VI stated it clearly in his encyclical *Humanae Vitae*. Pope John Paul II has made it clearer still, and referred to both Paul VI and the Council. On December 14, 1990, he called married couples to a sense of responsibility "for love and for life." This *responsibility*, the Pope makes clear, must guide them when they decide how many children they should have.

His words are so important they will be quoted here as reported in the English edition of *L'Osservatore Romano*: "Through this sense of responsibility for love and for life, God the Creator invites the spouses not to be passive operators, but rather 'cooperators or almost interpreters' of his plan (*Gaudium et Spes*, n. 50). In fact, they are called, out of respect for the objective moral order established by God, to an obligatory discernment of the indications of God's will concerning their family. Thus, in relationship to physical, economic, psychological and social conditions, responsible parenthood will be able to be expressed 'either by the deliberate and generous decision to raise a large family, or by the decision, made for serious moral reasons and with due respect for the moral law, to avoid for the time being, or even for an indeterminate period, another birth'" (*Humanae Vitae*, n. 10).

Pope John Paul II then goes on to caution against abusing NFP. He indicates that people must be taught its moral use so that they will see "it is not possible to practice natural methods as a 'licit' variation of the decision to be closed to life, which would be substantially the same as that which inspires the decision to use contraceptives: only if there is a basic openness to fatherhood and motherhood, understood as collaboration with the Creator, does the use of natural means become an integrating part of the responsibility for love and life."

Note that among the factors to be considered are "external conditions." In densely populated countries with a high population growth rate, a couple might meritoriously decide, for the common good, to have fewer children than they would like. But conversely, in nations which are not reproducing themselves, couples have an added responsibility to be generous in their decisions regarding family planning, in the name of God and country. Since in the U.S. the fertility rate has been below replacement level during most recent years, Fr. Paul Marx, O.S.B., of Human Life International, urges U.S. couples to plan their family, then plan one more.

The *Catechism of the Catholic Church* treats these same matters in a more general way. It says that the state can convey concerns and information regarding population matters, but it cannot "usurp the initiative of spouses" (n. 2372; see nn. 2366 to 2379).

Couples who respect God's law, themselves and their procreative powers enough to undertake the discipline of NFP are less likely to offend against responsible use of fertility. NFP makes them always aware of their power to procreate life. They may not be so generous as to bear more children than they feel is their duty in keeping with their marital "responsibility for life and for love," but they are not too likely to fall short of their duty.

Teachers who present NFP should also present the related human and spiritual values and responsibilities linked with it. Omitting the values that make it moral opens the way to abusing it. The natural methods are to be understood in the light of "the total vision of the human person and vocation, which is not only natural and earthly, but also supernatural and eternal," as Paul VI wrote in *Humanae Vitae* (n. 7).

Another abuse of NFP is to combine it with contraceptives during the fertile period, or to consummate the sexual act in other ways than intercourse. Such couples are really not using NFP; they are *only* abusing it. The rule is: abstinence during the fertile period, when the method is being used to exclude pregnancy.

15. But aren't there other reasons for not having children? Doesn't the population explosion justify contraception? Or the case of a young woman set on becoming a doctor and contributing to the miracle of modern medicine?

To answer both questions: the end does not justify the means. If the end is necessary, we can, in God's providence, discover a fit and moral means.

This is not a treatise on population, but the question here is asked as one related to family planning, so a few remarks on the topic could prove helpful. The fierce advocates of zero population growth are out of their depth. "Too many people!" is their cry. In his book, *Too Many People*, Christopher Derrick asks, "Too many for what?" For the state? For the security of the wealthy? He reminds all of us that forced population control is totalitarianism. The decision to procreate belongs in the hands of married couples, with whom God shares his prerogatives.

If people exist primarily for God, Derrick asks, how can you measure when there are "too many people"? He points out that the "population problem" is, at least in our time, quite different than too many people in any sense. It is, rather, the plurality of problems that arise with rapidly increasing population: provision of food, care of the environment, etc. These are real problems, but neither new nor insoluble. Population hysteria is the product of a myth created by population myth-makers.

These growth problems should be a concern of us all, but no reason for hysteria. Nor should they be allowed to rob married couples of the joy in their power to bear children, or in bearing them. Human beings are not products to be ordered by and produced for the state like guns and planes.

Our human dignity transcends that of the state, which is our servant, and which we will eternally outlast. When planning their family, couples should consider the common good. But they should never forget the good of the child to whom they can give life, and whom God can give eternal life. Nor does anyone have the right to cling to an affluent life style in such a way that he or she feels threatened by people, and creates population hysteria.

The "population explosion" is, in western countries, a population fizzle. Almost no western country has a birth rate adequate to avoid population shrinkage. Belgium, Denmark, France, Great Britain and Russia all have the problem. Germany's birth rate is about 70% of what is needed for a stable population.

In an address to bishops in October, 1985, Pope John Paul II said: "If the current demographic trend continues, the European population, which in 1960 constituted 25% of the world population, would by the middle of the next century drop to a level of 5%. These are figures that have led some European leaders to speak of the 'demographic suicide' of Europe."

For the U.S., *Statistical Abstracts 1984* reported the fertility rate from 1975-80 to be 6.3% *below* replacement level. If this continued, as the population ages it would shrink at the rate of 6.3% in a geometrical *degression*. There has been a slight rise in the birthrate in the U.S. during the first half of the 1990's, but it is only temporary. Women of the baby boom generation are having children just before they pass out of the child-bearing age, bringing the fertility rate in 1993 up to two children per woman per lifetime. But the fertility rate is projected to decline again soon, because the number of women in the child-bearing years is declining. In addition almost half of U.S. couples are sterile, mostly as a result of contraceptive sterilization.

Despite this less-than-replacement fertility rate in the U.S., the population has continued to grow for the present. This is due to immigration and also because good food and good health care are resulting in a temporary decline in the death rate. That rate will inevitably rise as the population grays.

Before we look at further trends, it will help to make three general statements about population that will enable the reader to better assess what has just been reported, and what follows: (1) Experience shows that population projections are unreliable, and constantly in need of revision; (2) While the birthrate is dangerously high in some countries, it is dangerously low in others; (3) This second factor cautions us that immoral means of reducing births can lead to graver problems than population growth itself.

India, China, Africa and Latin America have had serious problems of growing populations. But by 1982, the U.N.'s *Statistical Yearbook* was reporting that the rate of population increase was steadily dropping. It predicted that by 2110 the world population could stabilize at 10.5 billion people.

The FAO's Dr. Pawley estimated that, if necessary, the world food production could be increased to feed 36 billion people. That figure supports a statement of Pope John Paul II, who was echoing Paul VI: "Instead of increasing the amount of bread on the table of a hungry human race, as modern means of production are able to do today, there are thoughts of diminishing the number of those at the table through methods that are contrary to honesty."

Here are some trends since those 1980's figures: In April, 1992, the U.N. warned that the world's population would not peak at 10.5 billion people in 2110, but go on to peak at 11.5

billion in 2150. Yet by April 1993, China had, by "Draconian steps," reduced its fertility rate to 1.8 or 1.9 births per woman per lifetime (*New York Times,* 4/25/93, p. 1). That is well below replacement level in the long run, though China's population will continue to grow much larger for some years, because the ratio of young to old people is very large. What then of the future of Italy, which "has a birth rate of 1.29 children per woman of childbearing age." The Italian bishops assessed it as "the lowest birthrate among all the countries in the world" (*Catholic Standard and Times,* 11/18/93).

By March, 1994, in an article entitled "Climb in Russia's Death Rate Sets Off Population Implosion," the *New York Times* reported that the number of children born to each woman per lifetime has fallen from 2.17 only five years ago to slightly more than 1.4, and that the life expectancy of adult men "has plummeted to 60 years." The result is that "Russia faces an unusual population crisis that even optimists say will take a generation to reverse" (3/16/94, p. 1). In some African nations, AIDS is causing so many deaths that no one knows Africa's population future. India and many other countries still have serious problems of population growth to deal with. But in general, in the West, the birth rate is below that needed to sustain current population levels.

Look at the positive side of population growth. The immense progress in our time owes much to population growth. It has freed vast numbers of people to engage in the studies and research that have brought advances which have spread throughout the world. Among them is the green revolution that gives the world a surplus of food.

Warehouses in the U.S. and elsewhere are bulging with farm products that cannot be sold. Hunger in the world results not from a lack of food, but from inequity, greed, power struggles, war, indifference and other man-made evils.

NFP has the capacity to control population in the most moral, humane, family-centered way possible. Mother Teresa reports that her NFP program in India has reduced unwanted births by over one million. NFP, written large, is "honest" population control. (For further reflections on population issues, see the author's "The Proliferation of Population Problems," in *Why Humanae Vitae Was Right: A Reader*, edited by Janet E. Smith.)

The young woman who wants to contribute to the miracle of modern medicine should know about the child-spacing miracle of NFP. She should be reminded that what the world needs most is the miracle of men and women who, like Mother Teresa, bring the world many blessings by teaching it to live according to God's wisdom and will.

16. Does NFP put a strain on marriage?

Life is a strain. It is a struggle and an aspiration to growth and betterment. "Through many tribulations we must enter the kingdom of God" (Acts 14:22). If a couple is immature, undisciplined, unrealistic or just plain selfish, there will be strain.

A couple has to agree to the requirements of NFP. This involves sacrifice. Is that a strain? Clearly, it depends on the couple. It depends on their love, morality and religion—even their physical and psychological states.

Often, the wife fears that her husband will not agree to NFP. One doctor gave me his opinion: if the husband won't agree, the marriage is already in trouble.

NFP *can* ease the strain of marriage. Couples find peace in NFP's religious, moral, health, financial and aesthetic advantages. The husband who loves his wife, her body and her health finds devotion and closeness to her by living in harmony with her body's rhythms. The couple dedicated to God and his will and the good of society finds a special peace and joy in living fully attuned to the harmonies which the Creator has impressed upon creation.

Couples who are on the rebound from harmful methods are often more appreciative of NFP than newlyweds who have no idea of the blessing that has entered their lives.

Not strain but bliss comes to spouses who learn, during abstinence, to court one another all over again in the chaste ways of courtship. It keeps alive their whole relationship from the day they met. The rhythm of separating and uniting has been described by more than one couple as a cycle of courtships and honeymoons.

In a poll by Nona Aguilar, less than 1% of the NFP couples tabulated had been previously married and divorced, yet 70% had been married six years or more. These couples have certainly found some way of coping with strain. It may be NFP.

Our question comes down to this: Does sexual restraint put a strain on marriage? The honest answer seems to be that it is the best preservative of marriage.

In 1984, the feminist Germaine Greer revised her opinion of the sexual revolution. She now maintains that it duped women into thinking there was something wrong with them if they were not promiscuous, and so it encouraged them to "endanger their bodies" with contraceptives. She concluded that the sexual revolution has worsened the status of women.

Excerpts of her book in the *Sunday Times* of London provoked a flood of letters. But most agreed with her on one point: sexual restraint can enhance sexual pleasure.

The restraint required by NFP is a strain if not seen in a positive light. But couples who pay the cost as matter-of-factly as they pay their food and rent bills escape the strain.

Some fail to see NFP in an adequately positive light. One wife who practiced it for ten years admitted that it worked, it required only about ten days of abstinence, and it gave her peace of conscience. But she regretted and, it seems, resented its demands. Why not rather:

1) Accept reality. There is no painless family planning. Life has its burdens. Jesus told us we must carry our cross daily,

but with him the burden is light. The abstinence required by marital chastity may be for many the only cross or burden felt on a periodic basis and, therefore, a salutary reminder of their journey with Christ.

2) Accept cheerfully at least the unavoidable burdens of life. "God loves a cheerful giver" (2 Cor 9:7).

3) Be grateful for the best there is, the method which God, nature and devoted researchers and teachers have given us.

"Two men looked out through prison bars.

"The one saw mud, the other stars."

In the end there are two contrary attitudes among NFP users. The couples who have integrated sexuality into the wholesome wholeness of their love employ NFP as their servant. As masters of NFP they are pleased with their servant. The couple who fail to see intercourse as *part* of their love— who identify love with intercourse—see NFP as a domineering master. They may remain its slaves, but they will always nurse sullen resentment.

It is Nona Aguilar's insight that *intimacy* is the goal of romance. NFP leads to, cajoles, requires and inspires intimacy. Where it is achieved, it brings great rewards. Any strain occasioned by NFP is more than offset by the greater strains it dissolves.

17. NFP clearly takes a lot of motivation. Are there any advantages you have not mentioned?

So many positive points and fringe benefits of NFP are sprouting that we can't treat them all here. The Pope has stated that between contraception and NFP there is "a difference which is much wider and deeper than is usually thought, one which involves in the final analysis two irreconcilable concepts of the human person and of human sexuality."

From the vantage point of the reflections made so far, we

can gain a panoramic view of the advantages of NFP. NFP is not solely a human creation. It is a scientific discovery and plan that enables a couple to capitalize on the spiritual, intellectual, bodily, sexual nature of man and woman. It encourages these qualities to grow. It summons the husband to love and respect his wife by moderating the use of his ever-present fertility to combine with the waxing and waning of hers in the wisest fashion. The couple grow in intimate dialogue, mutual respect, shared responsibility and self control. They fuse and bond in a love that runs deep and tender.

NFP guides the couple along a way so harmonious to their nature that it does no harm to body or soul. It is graced with the moral and religious approval that suffuses them with peace of conscience. It enables them to escape the health and financial burden of drugs and devices. Women "feel liberated," says Dr. Hanna Klaus, when they learn there is fertility control without the pill.

Their intimate dialogue and practice of self control puts them so in tune with sex that they radiate a healthy attitude to their children. When it is time to instruct their children in the mysteries of sex, they do it with ease.

On planning to unite in the hope of conceiving a child, they can choose the time of highest fertility. They enter with heightened consciousness into union with God and one another to create life. *Let us make a human being like ourselves in God's image and likeness.*

If they conceive, they are apt to know the date as accurately as possible—no small advantage in planning for the day of delivery.

A woman becomes so knowledgeable about her cycle she is better able to monitor her health, and catch any disorders early. She comes to perceive the relationships of her mood changes to her menstrual cycle, predict them and plan to avoid stressful situations at her bad times. Her husband, privy to these alternations, adapts himself more considerately to her needs.

Times of abstinence become times to express love in tender

ways, times to return to the chaste expressions of courtship love. This journey back renews their whole love relationship. These non-selfish expressions of love are most dear to a woman. And what is appearing everywhere is that abstinence taken in stride is a boon to married love. It certainly eliminates boredom. "Abstinence," said one NFP user, "is the best aphrodisiac." It proves that romance doesn't belong only to the unmarried.

NFP intensifies each one's consciousness of his or her own body and the spouse's body. This heightens the relationship between between souls and bodies. This is especially true after a period of abstinence.

There is a nobility about NFP that should appeal in a special way to Christians, "zealous for good deeds" (Tit 2:14).

Low-fertility couples have the unique advantage of employing their knowledge of peak-fertility time to enhance their potential to have a child.

NFP has the singular advantage of being the full family planning method. Other methods plan only by prevention.

Even the sessions devoted to learning are rewarding. "Learning NFP," writes Fr. Richard Huneger, "is like taking a course in yourself."

NFP is the greatest enemy of abortion, the moral plague of our age. It enables couples to plan their family effectively. It does away with abortifacient devices like the IUD. If through weakness or, more rarely, the failure of the method, they have an unplanned child, another advantage is evident. The respect they have shown for the source of life instills such a reverence for life that it inspires them to change their plans and receive this child into their home with love. Thus NFP promoter Fr. Anthony Zimmerman looks with hope to "the post-abortion era of NFP."

NFP makes amends for another crime of our age: the attitudes that rob women, from girlhood on, of the joy of their sex. First, our age attacked and broke down sexual mores. Then it treated women with their power of motherhood as a threat to society. It became blind to seeing them for what they really are: the sole hope of any human future.

NFP creates a climate of respect for, and control of, human fertility. As it spreads, it will help rebuild our sexual mores, and our respect for the religions and religious authorities that fought so bravely to guard them. As Fr. Leo J. Shea, S.J. put it, NFP has the power to usher in "a bright new world of married love."

Perhaps all the advantages of NFP, known and unknown, are summed up in the statement of Pope John Paul II that "what is taught by the Church on responsible parenthood is none other than the original plan which the Creator imprinted on the humanity of the man and the woman who marry, and which the Redeemer came to reestablish." Who can conceive of a greater plus than that? It is nothing less than godlikeness.

As the years pass, we will discover more and more advantages of NFP. We have only begun.

18. You have referred repeatedly to the harm done by contraceptive methods. Would you elaborate?

Contraception suppresses the life-giving power of marital intercourse. This is its fundamental evil. The couple turn their act of total self-giving into dishonesty, turn to what is unnatural, and turn from God.

Some day a contraceptive may do no physical harm except to the person's fertility, but it will remain evil, and spawn evil. It degrades marriage and it diminishes the full personhood, the *embodiedness* of the spouses. By it, the body is used rather than respected in its own right, its own reality and its own fertility, which must not be "shoved out" of the relationship. However innocent the *intention* of users, using contraceptives demeans sex, distorts its meaning and contributes to the breakdown of sexual morality.

In *Humanae Vitae*, Pope Paul VI projected the consequences of accepting contraception: conjugal infidelity; the general lowering of morality; loss of manly respect for, and even concern for, a woman's physical and psychological equilibrium; and finally, government-forced contraception, as subsequently happened in India, and is happening in China.

Certainly, the sexual revolution, which was launched from the platform of contraception, has led to rampant divorce and recreational sex. These have led to a multiplication of single-parent families, which are coming to be seen as a poverty trap, a tragedy for children and mothers and a growing social burden.

Contraception is even an enemy of livelihood. The Couple to Couple League has estimated that over the fertile period of a woman's life, spouses can spend several thousand dollars for contraceptives. Add physician costs: 9.7 million visits involving family planning were made by U.S. women in one year (1977). Costs beyond this for health and other reasons are incalculable. Contrast this with NFP, which requires no doctors and costs almost nothing beyond the instruction stage.

Treating fertility as an enemy to be defeated demeans both men and women. The person who uses a contraceptive feels demeaned. The partner feels used. And they are.

Contraceptives lead to abortion. They dull respect for the source of human life, then for new human life, then for life itself. Planned Parenthood first promoted contraception as a means to avoid abortion; then abortion as backup contraception.

Pundits of Europe where all these evils flourished so riotously have now "proclaimed the 'death of man' as a person and transcendent value" as the Pope observed in October, 1985.

Contraceptives only too frequently are not really that at all. (Contraception means "against conception.") They work by aborting new life.

The pill is often an abortifacient as well. "The new, lower dosage pill," writes Dr. Herbert Ratner, "primarily interferes with the reproductive process at a late stage, ending pregnancy after an egg has been fertilized. Normally this new child implants itself in the wall of the uterus, where it will be protected and be able to nourish itself. But it can do this only if the uterus' wall (lining) has been made ready for the egg by a hormone sent from the ovary. The blocking of this hormone by the abortion agent prevents implantation by the tiny baby and ends pregnancy."

Berlin's drug firm Schering, the world's largest producer of female hormones, explains in its own literature that the pill works by hindering ovulation, by thickening cervical mucus to block sperm and by preventing the fertilized egg from implanting itself: "Given the content of the pill, the walls of the uterus do not properly develop, so that the embryo does not implant, or implants improperly."

Abortion used to be back-up contraception. Now it has moved to the front line. Already used in Europe, and now introduced in the U.S., is a prostaglandin-type chemical which will initiate abortion when used within thirty days of conception. It is designed to be taken once a month instead of the pill.

The IUD works by abortion. It also causes harmful side effects. In March, 1986, all major-sale IUD's were removed from the U.S. market because of the number of lawsuits by ailing women.

The pill was implicated in so much sickness and death that one warning after another was issued. Between 1973 and 1982 its use dropped by 44%.

Along with casual sex, contraceptives have contributed to the epidemic of herpes, gonorrhea, and other sexually-transmitted diseases.

Surgical sterilization, which was once a felony if used for birth control, has surged. By 1982, surgical sterilization had become the means of contraception for the wife or husband of 38.9% of fertility-age American couples. That so many have adopted such a drastic and often irreversible step testifies to the harm from other contraceptives.

On the question of the harm from the pill, let us hear Dr. Joseph Gambescia: "Not too long ago the beautiful tomato—the so called 'love apple'—was considered to be poisonous. It took an adventurous and curious person whose identity is lost to history to finally bite the tomato. Its nutritious and delicious character and flavor have ruled the roost these many years.

"Medical science today, with a number of guidelines (referred to collectively as the scientific method) avoids the necessity of the daring of our tomato pioneer. The scientific method is designed to accumulate sufficient data to evaluate proposed new treatments of whatever sort.

"Yet in the process of developing treatments and cures for humans, following a variety of experiments both *ex-vivo* and *in-vivo* in animals, there comes a time when a human person must be exposed to a new diagnostic or therapeutic modality. This could be by self-experimentation, by the use of volunteers—and in certain instances the use of controls—and, of course, by individuals who have not responded to other forms of therapy.

"In 1965 and again in 1974, the World Health Organization compiled a series of principles: the Helsinki Declaration. It was designed to safeguard the health of those individuals involved in the process of human experimentation by one means or another. The presumption was that the health of the patient was the first consideration for the doctor. The declaration separated distinctly medical research, in which the aim is essentially therapeutic or diagnostic, from medical research which has a purely scientific aim with no direct diagnostic and therapeutic benefits.

"I often wonder whether, if these principles had been firmly in place, the oral contraceptives as they were introduced in the U.S. in the 1960's would have been accepted. To me it seemed to be a big experiment, foisted on the American public, particularly the women of America. It was touted as a great panacea, yet hidden within it as within a Pandora's box, a host of asp-like problems lay in wait ready to strike. There were heart disease, hypertension, stroke, thrombosis, liver tumors—to say nothing of nausea, vomiting, headache and depression. Since their introduction, the list of adverse effects has become longer and longer. The space in *The Physicians Desk Reference* devoted to warnings and adverse reactions becomes greater and greater. As a matter of fact, the original formulation in great measure has been changed, but the adverse reactions increase in type and number. Indeed, it was a big experiment, and we continue to collect data in this experiment, as evidenced by the medical literature devoted to warnings about it.

"We are much involved in countering the pollution of our environment, and rightly so. Why do we permit the pollution of our internal environment—our body—to treat a non-disease?

"It is hoped that the medical community will soon awaken to this schizophrenic approach, and remove itself from the advocacy of drugs and devices which treat no illness but cause illness of themselves."

It is no wonder, then, that the pill has driven people to seek other forms of birth control. But neither are other forms of contraception the answer. They all have their own problems, whether to morals or to health, or to both. Certainly, sterilization is a serious moral evil. In *Humanae Vitae*, Paul VI stated this clearly. Having absolutely condemned abortion, he added: "Equally to be excluded, as the teaching authority of the Church has frequently declared, is direct sterilization, whether perpetual or temporary, whether of the man or the woman."

The devastating effects of contraception and abortion on whole populations was referred to in question fifteen. No one yet knows what future evils of this kind they may bring about if NFP does not displace them with its pro-life mentality.

All of this has dealt a grievous wound to religion. The Catholic Church condemns both abortion and contraception. (Until 1930, so did other Christian churches. See John Kippley's booklet, *Birth Control and Christian Discipleship*.) In consequence, many have fallen away from the Church. Many have remained, but also remained at odds with their pastors; or both laity and pastors have rejected the teaching of the Pope and the bishops.

The gravity of this comes home only if we remember that God alone is *he who knows*, and that we know in matters of faith only by faith. The harm done by contraceptives cannot be seen in its fullness until we recall that we must all one day stand for judgment before the Lord, and accept the consequences of our deeds.

NFP is the providential gift of God to heal many of these wounds. Anyone who contributes to its spread by prayer of petition, by teaching it or setting the example of using it, or making badly needed financial contributions to NFP organizations, does a loving work of great compassion. The suffering and anguish of many will be alleviated if they come to know NFP in its true meaning and efficacy.

19. Where can I learn more? And if I decide in favor, where can I learn NFP?

To learn more, *read*. A book that masterfully treats many aspects of NFP is John and Sheila Kippley's *The Art Of Natural Family Planning*. If you are particularly interested in the experiences of couples, enjoy Nona Aguilar's *No Pill—No Risk Birth Control*. For a book that ranges more into spiritual aspects, see *Challenge to Love* by Mary Shivanandan. A wide-ranging treatment of OM will be found in Mercedes Arzu Wilson's *The Ovulation Method of Birth Regulation*. Manuals directed to learning the actual use of NFP can begin with *The Ovulation Method* by John Billings, M.D. It is a brief, lucid description of OM by its most exhaustive researcher.

For a thorough treatment of the Sympto-Thermal Method, there is Dr. Josef Roetzer's excellent *Family Planning The Natural Way*. His treatment has been boiled down to a client's manual in *Comprehensive Fertility Awareness And Natural Family Planning*, by Fr. Richard J. Huneger. There is also the Kippley book recommended above. Another clear, brief presentation of STM can be found in *The Double-Check Method of Family Planning* by Paul Thyma.

Natural Family Planning: A Review, by Hanna Klaus, M.D., is an invaluable technical overview of the subject suited to doctors and professionals in the field.

From the religious, theological and moral vantage point, the outstanding treatment remains Pope Paul VI's encyclical *Humanae Vitae*. It is brief and prophetic. Pope John Paul II has added a valuable updated commentary in *Reflections On Humanae Vitae*. John Kippley ranges over the whole issue of contraception and NFP in *Sex And The Marriage Covenant.*

Pope John Paul II provides some profound observations and directives on NFP in *The Role Of The Christian Family In The Modern World*. In *A Theological Perspective On NFP*, Msgr. James T. McHugh theologizes on the subject. In *Why Humanae Vitae Was Right: A Reader*, Janet E. Smith gives us what James Hitchcock calls "a superb collection of articles on every aspect of the encyclical and the issues that followed from it."

These books are listed in the book list that follows.

To learn to use NFP, contact reliable and well-trained teachers. Phone the Catholic Chancery closest to you (listed in your phone book in large cities), request the Family Life Bureau, and ask how to enroll in an NFP course. Such programs are open to all comers without religious requirements. The brief courses (one to four sessions) are usually taught by NFP user-couples. From a background of experience they provide instruction, assurance and support.

Try your nearest Catholic hospital. They may have a program. Or ask your Catholic pastor. He can direct you to the diocesan program, and it's good to get him involved in this movement.

Diocesan programs usually teach both OM and STM. If you would like to learn NFP in a way that focuses on OM, contact the Family of the Americas Foundation, or the NFP Center of Washington, D.C., or the Paul VI Institute for the Study of Human Reproduction (see the *List of Providers* given further on).

If a diocese does not have a program, or has one that a couple is not satisfied with, in looking elsewhere the couple should seek out a program that includes value orientation, and that does not combine NFP with contraceptives during the fertile period—a tactic which corrupts its moral meaning, and lowers its effectiveness. Among the independent organizations that can be relied on for this is the Couple to Couple League. Co-founded by John and Sheila Kippley and Dr. Konald A. Prem, CCL is devoted to teaching NFP directly through a network of trained couples throughout the country. It publishes the bi-monthly *CCL Family Foundations*, "to keep couples up-to-date in NFP, and offer support." The publication is a gold mine.

The Couple to Couple League has a home-study course for people who live in regions where they have no access to NFP programs or teachers. The league believes this is a significant advance over the use of any book. For information about the availability of NFP classes in your area, or the home study course and materials, contact the Couple to Couple League.

One way to find information locally is simply for couples to mention in casual conversations that they have heard good things about NFP. They may find that a couple will speak out enthusiastically about NFP, or at least approach them privately and steer them to help, and even offer to answer questions if the inquirers should adopt NFP.

User-couples who thank God for the method should think of thanking him in the practical way of volunteering as teacher couples. Contact any of the teaching sources just mentioned. You will receive teacher training. Couples owe this to God and one another. "Couples helping couples" is an NFP watchword.

"Lift up your eyes, and see how the fields are already white for harvest" (Jn. 4:35). "Laborers are few; pray therefore the Lord of the harvest to send out laboreres into his harvest" (Mt. 9:37). Beg him to send you. This harvest master pays wages beyond your wildest dreams.

"Now is the day of salvation" (2 Cor 6:2). Any one of these books, addresses, or phone numbers *put to use* is the first step to the very best in family planning.

NATIONAL AND REGIONAL NFP PROVIDERS

(For updates of this list, contact the Diocesan Development Program for Natural Family Planning, 3211 4th St. N.E., Washington, DC 20017-1194, 202-541-3240).

Billings Ovulation Method Association, Hanna Klaus, M.D., Director, 8514 Bradmoor Dr., Bethesda, MD 20817 (301-897-9323).

Centro Billings de Los Angeles, Alejandro and Lilia Morelos, Coordinators, 933 S. Grattan St., Los Angeles, CA 90015 (213-251-3214).

The Couple to Couple League, John Kippley, President, P.O. Box 111184, Cincinnati, OH 45211 (513-471-2000).

Family of the Americas Foundation, Mercedes Wilson, Executive Director, P.O. Box 1170, Dunkirk, MD 20754 (301-627-3346).

Family Life Promotion of New York, Carman and Jean Fallace, Directors, P.O. Box 115, Lake Grove, NY 11755 (516-981-1971).

Natural Family Planning of the Alleghenies, Rosemarie Kieswetter, Director, 3300 Beale Ave., Altoona, PA 16601 (814-946-3544).

Natural Family Planning of Greater Kansas City, Inc., Phyllis White, Director, P.O. Box 24703, Kansas City, MO 64131 (816-765-5866).

Northwest Family Services, Inc., Rose Fuller, Executive Director, 4805 N.E. Glisan St., Portland, OR 97213 (503-230-6377).

Paul VI Institute for the Study of Human Reproduction, Thomas Hilgers, M.D., Executive Director, 6901 Mercy Rd., Omaha, NE 68106 (402-390-6600).

Twin Cities NFP Center, Inc., Don Kramer, Director, Health East St. Joseph's Hospital, 69 W. Exchange St., St. Paul, MN 55102-1053 (612-232-3088).

"What Every Woman Should Know" Outreach Program-USA, June E. Frakes, R.N., and Roy E. Frakes Coordinators, P.O. Box 41, Wofford Heights, CA 93285-0041 (619-376-3850).

WOOMB Bilingual-Bicultural, Patricia Pointdexter, R.N., Director, 7532 East Cecilia St., Downey, CA 90241 (310-928-4433).

BOOKLIST

A good number of the publications listed below are available through any of the Pauline Book & Media Centers listed at the end of this booklet, or from the Couple to Couple League, P.O. Box 111184, Cincinnati, OH 45211 (513-471-2000). Contact them for a catalog. Out-of-print books may be available through inter-library loan.

The Art of Natural Family Planning. John and Sheila Kippley.

The Best of Natural Family Planning. ed: Rev. Paul Marx, O.S.B.

Birth Control and Christian Discipleship. John Kippley.

The Billings Method, Controlling Fertility Without Drugs or Devices. Dr. Evelyn Billings and Ann Westmore.

Breast Feeding And Natural Child Spacing. Sheila Kippley.

CCL Home Study Course (A complete home course on Natural Family Planning). The Couple to Couple League.

Challenge to Love. Mary Shivanandan.

Comprehensive Fertility Awareness & NFP (Client Assignments). Richard Huneger

Double Check Method Of Family Planning. Paul Thyma.

Family Planning The Natural Way. Josef Roetzer, M.D.

History of the Biologic Control of Human Fertility. Jan Mucharski.

Humanae Vitae, On The Regulation Of Births. Pope Paul VI.

Joy Of Being A Woman. Ingrid Trobisch.

Know Your Body, A Family Guide To Sexuality And Fertility. Charles W. Norris, M.D. and J. B. W. Owen.

Natural Family Planning: A review. Dr. Hanna Klaus.

Natural Family Planning, The Ovulation Method. John Billings, M.D.

Natural Family Planning, Nature's Way, God's Way. ed: Fr. Anthony Zimmerman *et al.*

The New No Pill—No Risk Birth Control. Nona Aguilar.

The Ovulation Method Of Birth Regulation. Mercedes Arzu Wilson.

Reflections On Humanae Vitae. Pope John Paul II.

The Role Of The Christian Family In The Modern World (Familiaris Consortio). Pope John Paul II.

Sex and the Marriage Covenant. John Kippley.

A Theological Perspective On Natural Family Planning. Msgr. James T. McHugh, S.T.D.

Why Humanae Vitae Was Right: A Reader. ed: Janet E. Smith.

ABOUT THE AUTHOR

An internationally published author of spiritual and theological works, and a veteran retreat master, Fr. Smith is regional director and Philadelphia Archdiocesan director of the Apostleship of Prayer.

More recent among his dozen books and numerous articles are the books *Sunday Homilies; Prayer and Personality Development; Homosexuality: The Questions* (co-authored); *Hidden Victory: A Historical Novel of Jesus;* and *Pro-Choice? Pro-Life? The Questions, The Answers.*

Fr. Smith is an occasional guest speaker on International Sacred Heart Radio. For some years he hosted the Spiritual Exercises Of the Air, a weekly radio program in greater Philadelphia. This long-running series included some 30 programs on natural family planning. They involved him in interviews with a number of prominent world, national and regional figures in natural family planning, including Fr. Paul Marx, O.S.B., Mercedes Wilson, Dr. Claude Lanctot, Dr. Josef Roetzer, John Kippley, Dr. Hanna Klaus, Jeff Spieler, Larry Kane, Fr. Richard Huneger, Nona Aguilar, Fr. Anthony Zimmerman, Dr. Sr. Catherine Bernard, Dr. Charles W. Norris, Dr. Kwang-ho Meng, Fr. Marc Caligari, S.J., Mary Shivanandan, Monsignor (now Bishop) James T. McHugh, and Ingrid Trobisch.

Fr. Smith offers to conduct days of recollection for NFP teachers and users, and to help them found a section of the Apostleship of Prayer for NFP teachers and users: *The Natural Family Planning League of the Sacred Heart.* He believes it will call down the divine intercession that will bless teachers and users, and help them awaken the Catholic population and the world to the family-healing and society-healing value of NFP.

Fr. Smith is a member of the Fellowship of Catholic Scholars. He resides in the Jesuit Community at Saint Joseph's University in Philadelphia.

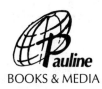

BOOKS & MEDIA

The Daughters of St. Paul operate book and media centers at the following addresses. Visit, call or write the one nearest you today, or find us on the World Wide Web, www.pauline.org

CALIFORNIA
  3908 Sepulveda Blvd., Culver City, CA 90230; 310-397-8676
  5945 Balboa Ave., San Diego, CA 92111; 619-565-9181
  46 Geary Street, San Francisco, CA 94108; 415-781-5180

FLORIDA
  145 S.W. 107th Ave., Miami, FL 33174; 305-559-6715

HAWAII
  1143 Bishop Street, Honolulu, HI 96813; 808-521-2731
  Neighbor Islands call: 800-259-8463

ILLINOIS
  172 North Michigan Ave., Chicago, IL 60601; 312-346-4228

LOUISIANA
  4403 Veterans Memorial Blvd., Metairie, LA 70006; 504-887-7631

MASSACHUSETTS
  Rte. 1, 885 Providence Hwy., Dedham, MA 02026; 781-326-5385

MISSOURI
  9804 Watson Rd., St. Louis, MO 63126; 314-965-3512

NEW JERSEY
  561 U.S. Route 1, Wick Plaza, Edison, NJ 08817; 732-572-1200

NEW YORK
  150 East 52nd Street, New York, NY 10022; 212-754-1110
  78 Fort Place, Staten Island, NY 10301; 718-447-5071

OHIO
  2105 Ontario Street, Cleveland, OH 44115; 216-621-9427

PENNSYLVANIA
  9171-A Roosevelt Blvd., Philadelphia, PA 19114; 215-676-9494

SOUTH CAROLINA
  243 King Street, Charleston, SC 29401; 843-577-0175

TENNESSEE
  4811 Poplar Ave., Memphis, TN 38117; 901-761-2987

TEXAS
  114 Main Plaza, San Antonio, TX 78205; 210-224-8101

VIRGINIA
  1025 King Street, Alexandria, VA 22314; 703-549-3806

CANADA
  3022 Dufferin Street, Toronto, Ontario, Canada M6B 3T5; 416-781-9131
  1155 Yonge Street, Toronto, Ontario, Canada M4T 1W2; 416-934-3440

¡También somos su fuente para libros, videos y música en español!